Survey of College Health Services: COVID Testing Practices

AF877988

ISBN 978-1-57440-701-3 ©2021 Primary Research Group Inc.

Table of Contents

THE QUESTIONNAIRE

1. Provide the following information:

A. Name
B. Title
C. Institution
D. Email Address

2. Your college or university is public or private

A. Public
B. Private

3. Your college or university is best described as:

A. Junior College
B. BA-Granting
C. MA or PHD Granting
D. Research University

4. What is your college/university's total approximate FTE enrollment for all schools and programs?

5. What is the average annual price of undergraduate tuition, the so-called sticker price, before financial aid or deductions?

6. How would you best describe your college's current operating model?

A. Completely or nearly completely remote learning based
B. Mostly online with some in-person classes
C. Mostly in-person classes
D. Completely or nearly completely in person classes

7. Does the college/university conduct wastewater testing as one way for assessing COVID risks?

A. Yes
B. No

8. What is the colleges' current test positivity rate?

9. Does the college conduct random testing of students to help monitor the potential for outbreaks?

A. Yes
B. No

10. Did the college require a pre- move-in COVID test for students who plan to live on campus?

A. Yes
B. No

11. If you college outsources COVID testing what are the names of your providers and how much are you paying per test?

12. How often are student athletes tested at your institution and how does their testing regime differ from that of other students?

13. What is the one or two major changes that you would make in your college's COVID control and prevention regime?

Time Frame of Surveying:

8/31/2021 10/4/2021

PARTICIPANT LIST

Aquinas College
Arkansas Tech University
Bucknell University
California State Polytechnic University
California State University Long Beach
Duquesne University
Florida Atlantic University
Henderson State University
Illinois College
Indiana University
Miles College
Mount Royal University
Napa Valley College
Northern Kentucky University
Northwest Missouri State University
Occidental College
Ohlone College
PCC
Princeton University
Texas Tech University Student Health Services
The New School
University of New Hampshire
University of New Hampshire
University of Wyoming
USD Wellness Center
Washington State University
Wayne State College

Characteristics of the sample

Public or private college

	#
Public	21
Private	9
Total	30

Type or carnegie class

	#
Junior College	4
BA-Granting	10
MA or PHD Granting	6
Research University	10
Total	30

FTE enrolment

	#
Less than 5000	9
5000+ - 10000	5
10000+ - 15000	8
More than 15000	8
Total	30

Tuition, $ USD

	#
Less than $8000	10
$8000+ - $15000	6
$15000+ - $30000	6
More than $30000	8
Total	30

Current operating model

	#
Completely or nearly completely remote learning based	0
Mostly online with some in-person classes	6
Mostly in-person classes	14
Completely or nearly completely in person classes	10
Total	30

% of students in college-provided dormitories

	#
Less than 10%	6
10% + - 30%	8
30% + - 60%	8
More than 60%	8
Total	30

SUMMARY OF MAIN FINDING

Use of Wastewater Testing

We asked: Does the college/university conduct wastewater testing as a way for assessing for COVID risks?

Only 13.33% of colleges surveyed tested wastewater to identify possible clusters of COVID on campus. All use was by research universities of which 40% in the sample used wastewater testing.

Current Test Positivity Rate

We asked: What is the college's current test positivity rate (for COVID)?

The mean was 8.03% (shockingly high!) though the median was 3.75%, nonetheless concerning. Positivity was much higher at public than private colleges; at public colleges it was 10.02% and even the median was a concerning 9% while for private colleges the rage was only 2.08% for the mean and 1.81% for the median. If American public colleges and universities were an independent country, it is likely that the US Government would seek to restrict the citizens of this College State from traveling to the USA and it would issue stern warnings to American citizens who wanted to visit the troubled, COVID-ridden country. The fact that the median is quite high is particularly concerning as widespread COVID does not appear to be mostly a factor of a few outliers driving up the overall mean. The spread is broad and the problem not restricted only to a handful of problem children.

For whatever reasons, MA/PHD granting institutions in the sample had particularly high rates while research universities had particularly low rates. The mean rate at research universities was 2.74% while the median rate was 1.5%, quite tolerable. However, for the MA/PHD granting institutions the mean was 19.03% and even the median an intolerable and dangerous 17.5%.

Moreover, rates were low at any college charging more than $15,000 per year in annual tuition. Under this level, the situation is far more precarious, even abjectly dangerous. Generally, many public colleges and universities in the USA are not safe environments for older or immune compromised individuals who are not vaccinated. This appears to be especially true for public research-oriented institutions that are not research universities. Perhaps these colleges have dormitories and extended PHD and graduate programs that involve greater risk than common at colleges that serve only a local community in a limited way. However, while they have more dormitories and greater need for interaction than local colleges, they do not have the resources to offer the protection common at the more celebrated, full research institutions, of which even the public variety are often state flagships and well- funded.

Use of Random Testing

We asked: Does the college conduct random testing of students to help monitor the potential for outbreaks?

Only 30% of colleges in the sample did so. It was far more common among private than public colleges; 44.44% of the former but only 23.81% of the latter conducted random tests. MA or PHD granting colleges, which in our sample had very high COVID positivity rates, did no such testing at all, an urgent need in this population. This kind of random testing was most common at colleges at which more than 60% of students lived in college dorms, but colleges with smaller populations in dorms, but lacking the will or awareness to conduct needed testing, may be the bigger problem here. For example, 62.5% of colleges with more than 60% of their students living in dorms conducted random tests but only 12.5% of colleges with between 10% and 60% of their students in dorms conducted such testing.

Requirements for Pre-Move-In Tests for Students Living on Campus

We asked: Did the college require a pre-move-in COVID test for students who plan to live on campus?

30% of colleges required such a pre move in COVID test. Once again, private colleges were much more aggressive than public ones; 55.56% of the former required pre move in COVID tests vs only 19.05% of public colleges.

Names of Providers for Outsourced Tests

We asked: If your college outsources COVID testing what are the names of your providers and how much are you paying per test?

A range of providers listed.

We asked: How often are student athletes tested at your institution and how does their testing regime differ from that of other students?

For many it was weekly; for some two or three times per week, particularly when a sport is in season. Policies sometimes differed for the vaccinated and unvaccinated and for some colleges no special arrangements existed for college athletes.

We asked: What is the one or two major changes that you would make in your college's COVID control and prevention regime?

Generally, more and more effective mandates for masking and vaccines. Also, controls on events at which alcohol is consumed and more and better screening and testing.

Table 1.1 Does the college/university conduct wastewater testing as one way for assessing COVID risks?

	No Answer	Yes	No
Entire sample	10.00%	13.33%	76.67%

Table 1.2 Does the college/university conduct wastewater testing as one way for assessing COVID risks? Broken out by public or private college

Public or private college	No Answer	Yes	No
Public	9.52%	14.29%	76.19%
Private	11.11%	11.11%	77.78%

Table 1.3 Does the college/university conduct wastewater testing as one way for assessing COVID risks? Broken out by type or carnegie class

Type or carnegie class	No Answer	Yes	No
Junior College	0.00%	0.00%	100.00%
BA-Granting	20.00%	0.00%	80.00%
MA or PHD Granting	0.00%	0.00%	100.00%
Research University	10.00%	40.00%	50.00%

Table 1.4 Does the college/university conduct wastewater testing as one way for assessing COVID risks? Broken out by FTE enrollment

FTE enrollment	No Answer	Yes	No
Less than 5000	11.11%	0.00%	88.89%
5000+ - 10000	0.00%	20.00%	80.00%
10000+ - 15000	25.00%	25.00%	50.00%
More than 15000	0.00%	12.50%	87.50%

Table 1.5 Does the college/university conduct wastewater testing as one way for assessing COVID risks? Broken out by tuition, $ USD

Tuition, $ USD	No Answer	Yes	No
Less than $8000	0.00%	0.00%	100.00%
$8000+ - $15000	33.33%	16.67%	50.00%
$15000+ - $30000	16.67%	33.33%	50.00%
More than $30000	0.00%	12.50%	87.50%

Table 1.6 Does the college/university conduct wastewater testing as one way for assessing COVID risks? Broken out by current operating model

Current operating model	No Answer	Yes	No
Mostly online with some in-person classes	0.00%	0.00%	100.00%
Mostly in-person classes	21.43%	7.14%	71.43%
Completely or nearly completely in person classes	0.00%	30.00%	70.00%

Table 1.7 Does the college/university conduct wastewater testing as one way for assessing COVID risks? Broken out by % of students in college-provided dormitories

% of students in college-provided dormitories	No Answer	Yes	No
Less than 10%	0.00%	0.00%	100.00%
10% + - 30%	12.50%	12.50%	75.00%
30% + - 60%	25.00%	12.50%	62.50%
More than 60%	0.00%	25.00%	75.00%

Table 2.1 What is the colleges' current test positivity rate?

	Mean	Median	Minimum	Maximum
Entire sample	8.03	3.75	0.20	40.00

Table 2.2 What is the colleges' current test positivity rate? Broken out by public or private college

Public or private college	Mean	Median	Minimum	Maximum
Public	10.02	9.00	0.20	40.00
Private	2.08	1.81	0.21	4.50

Table 2.3 What is the colleges' current test positivity rate? Broken out by type or carnegie class

Type or carnegie class	Mean	Median	Minimum	Maximum
Junior College	5.50	5.50	1.00	10.00
BA-Granting	6.25	6.25	2.50	10.00
MA or PHD Granting	19.03	17.50	1.11	40.00
Research University	2.74	1.50	0.20	10.00

Table 2.4 What is the colleges' current test positivity rate? Broken out by FTE enrollment

FTE enrollment	Mean	Median	Minimum	Maximum
Less than 5000	8.60	4.50	1.00	25.00
5000+ - 10000	4.83	4.56	0.21	10.00
10000+ - 15000	1.40	1.00	0.20	3.00
More than 15000	15.50	10.00	2.00	40.00

Table 2.5 What is the colleges' current test positivity rate? Broken out by tuition, $ USD

Tuition, $ USD	Mean	Median	Minimum	Maximum
Less than $8000	6.00	6.50	1.00	10.00
$8000+ - $15000	20.75	17.50	8.00	40.00
$15000+ - $30000	0.60	0.60	0.20	1.00
More than $30000	2.08	1.81	0.21	4.50

Table 2.6 What is the colleges' current test positivity rate? Broken out by current operating model

Current operating model	Mean	Median	Minimum	Maximum
Mostly online with some in-person classes	4.33	2.00	1.00	10.00
Mostly in-person classes	10.93	8.00	1.00	40.00
Completely or nearly completely in person classes	6.50	1.81	0.20	25.00

Table 2.7 What is the colleges' current test positivity rate? Broken out by % of students in college-provided dormitories

% of students in college-provided dormitories	Mean	Median	Minimum	Maximum
Less than 10%	4.33	2.00	1.00	10.00
10% + - 30%	12.02	9.00	1.11	40.00
30% + - 60%	12.00	10.00	1.00	25.00
More than 60%	1.85	1.36	0.20	4.50

Table 3.1 Does the college conduct random testing of students to help monitor the potential for outbreaks?

	No Answer	Yes	No
Entire sample	10.00%	30.00%	60.00%

Table 3.2 Does the college conduct random testing of students to help monitor the potential for outbreaks? Broken out by public or private college

Public or private college	No Answer	Yes	No
Public	9.52%	23.81%	66.67%
Private	11.11%	44.44%	44.44%

Table 3.3 Does the college conduct random testing of students to help monitor the potential for outbreaks? Broken out by type or carnegie class

Type or carnegie class	No Answer	Yes	No
Junior College	0.00%	50.00%	50.00%
BA-Granting	20.00%	30.00%	50.00%
MA or PHD Granting	0.00%	0.00%	100.00%
Research University	10.00%	40.00%	50.00%

Table 3.4 Does the college conduct random testing of students to help monitor the potential for outbreaks? Broken out by FTE enrollment

FTE enrollment	No Answer	Yes	No
Less than 5000	11.11%	22.22%	66.67%
5000+ - 10000	0.00%	40.00%	60.00%
10000+ - 15000	25.00%	37.50%	37.50%
More than 15000	0.00%	25.00%	75.00%

Table 3.5 Does the college conduct random testing of students to help monitor the potential for outbreaks? Broken out by tuition, $ USD

Tuition, $ USD	No Answer	Yes	No
Less than $8000	0.00%	30.00%	70.00%
$8000+ - $15000	33.33%	0.00%	66.67%
$15000+ - $30000	16.67%	33.33%	50.00%
More than $30000	0.00%	50.00%	50.00%

Table 3.6 Does the college conduct random testing of students to help monitor the potential for outbreaks? Broken out by current operating model

Current operating model	No Answer	Yes	No
Mostly online with some in-person classes	0.00%	33.33%	66.67%
Mostly in-person classes	21.43%	21.43%	57.14%
Completely or nearly completely in person classes	0.00%	40.00%	60.00%

Table 3.7 Does the college conduct random testing of students to help monitor the potential for outbreaks? Broken out by % of students in college-provided dormitories

% of students in college-provided dormitories	No Answer	Yes	No
Less than 10%	0.00%	33.33%	66.67%
10% + - 30%	12.50%	12.50%	75.00%
30% + - 60%	25.00%	12.50%	62.50%
More than 60%	0.00%	62.50%	37.50%

Table 4.1 Did the college require a pre- move-in COVID test for students who plan to live on campus?

	No Answer	Yes	No
Entire sample	13.33%	30.00%	56.67%

Table 4.2 Did the college require a pre- move-in COVID test for students who plan to live on campus? Broken out by public or private college

Public or private college	No Answer	Yes	No
Public	14.29%	19.05%	66.67%
Private	11.11%	55.56%	33.33%

Table 4.3 Did the college require a pre- move-in COVID test for students who plan to live on campus? Broken out by type or carnegie class

Type or carnegie class	No Answer	Yes	No
Junior College	25.00%	0.00%	75.00%
BA-Granting	20.00%	30.00%	50.00%
MA or PHD Granting	0.00%	50.00%	50.00%
Research University	10.00%	30.00%	60.00%

Table 4.4 Did the college require a pre- move-in COVID test for students who plan to live on campus? Broken out by FTE enrollment

FTE enrollment	No Answer	Yes	No
Less than 5000	22.22%	44.44%	33.33%
5000+ - 10000	0.00%	20.00%	80.00%
10000+ - 15000	25.00%	12.50%	62.50%
More than 15000	0.00%	37.50%	62.50%

Table 4.5 Did the college require a pre- move-in COVID test for students who plan to live on campus? Broken out by tuition, $ USD

Tuition, $ USD	No Answer	Yes	No
Less than $8000	10.00%	20.00%	70.00%
$8000+ - $15000	33.33%	0.00%	66.67%
$15000+ - $30000	16.67%	33.33%	50.00%
More than $30000	0.00%	62.50%	37.50%

Table 4.6 Did the college require a pre- move-in COVID test for students who plan to live on campus? Broken out by current operating model

Current operating model	No Answer	Yes	No
Mostly online with some in-person classes	16.67%	33.33%	50.00%
Mostly in-person classes	21.43%	21.43%	57.14%
Completely or nearly completely in person classes	0.00%	40.00%	60.00%

Table 4.7 Did the college require a pre- move-in COVID test for students who plan to live on campus? Broken out by % of students in college-provided dormitories

% of students in college-provided dormitories	No Answer	Yes	No
Less than 10%	16.67%	16.67%	66.67%
10% + - 30%	12.50%	12.50%	75.00%
30% + - 60%	25.00%	37.50%	37.50%
More than 60%	0.00%	50.00%	50.00%

If your college outsources COVID testing what are the names of your providers and how much are you paying per test?

Less than 10% of students live on campus in dormitories/suites.

1) Our university is carrying the cost of the rapid testing program on campus. I don't know the costs of this.
2) Test free
3) Virusgeeks insurance is charged / billed
4) ShieldT3

10% + - 30%

1) Binx cost unknown
2) Arkansas Dept of Health; university has state funding provided for testing
3) Incyte, they are also billing the students. Unknown what this contract cost. Also, student health employees are testing students.
4) TDEM and free
5) testing largely on campus
6) N/A
7) In-house

30% + - 60%

1) Providence Medical Center 100.00 each
2) No
3) Unsure
4) FloMedi
5) N/A

More than 60%

1) Genetworx
2) Unknown
3) Genetworx $65
4) N/A, testing done on campus
5) N/A
6) N/A

Less than 10%

1) I don't believe that there is a testing regime for student athletes
2) Weekly
3) Athletes required to get baseline PCR; thereafter only non-vaccinated students are required to test. They are tested weekly. Other students are similar -- weekly testing for non-vaccinated people, but no baseline test is required.
4) Not sure
5) Weekly and yes

10% + - 30%

1) N/A
2) Not sure- they do surveillance but unsure how often; this is conducted by the Athletic Training staff
3) Probably daily. Other students must be symptomatic to get tested
4) 3X per week
5) Several times weekly; main population only if symptomatic or listed as contact
6) Twice a week if in season regular students not tested unless they request it
7) Weekly to monthly

30% + - 60%

1) Same as students Univac 2 times a week, vac one time every other week
2) 3x per week for unvaccinated
3) Same as everyone else
4) Tested, if don't have a card (proof of Shot)
5) 1x/week, yes
6) Weekly

More than 60%

1) Unsure
2) Once a week
3) Only unvaccinated and once weekly, same as the rest of the students
4) According to NCAA
5) Once a week for all vaccinated students, twice a week for non-vaccinated
6) Same; twice weekly if unvaccinated; every 2 weeks if vaccinated

Less than 10%

1) Mandated vaccinations
2) Not necessary outside of increasing vaccinated groups
3) We currently mandate vaccination for only a small number of in-person classes. I would favor a mandate for all in-person classes.
4) Enforcement and consequences

10% + - 30%

1) More social distancing, more space for isolation and a larger contact tracing team separate from Student Health Services
2) Require vaccines for all state universities
3) Send a message to faculty and students that nobody should be attending class or freely walk the campus while sick. If students are sick, they should be given a Zoom link to attend class that way. Professors need to be more lenient. WSU needs to be more proactive and less reactive.
4) Masks required
5) Better control of off-campus events and gatherings
6) Require vaccination, not have housing at full capacity
7) More testing better mask compliance better enforcement

30% + - 60%

1) Ability to mandate vaccination better use of masks
2) Enforce masks during class, Mandatory vaccines
3) More labor force
4) Mask mandate, social distancing mandate, more virtual class options
5) More online class offerings, social distancing and enforce masking policy

More than 60%

1) Better communication, not so many people involved in reporting process.
2) Do more online classes
3) Larger contact tracing team
4) Allowing the clinical departments (health majors) to self-conduct asymptomatic screenings.
5) Ban alcohol events which cause congregation and punish those who do not comply
6) Indoor mask mandate for all indoor spaces, not just classrooms. No outside campus visitors.

Made in United States
North Haven, CT
05 November 2026